Copyright © 2007 by Bramcost Publications
All rights reserved
Published in the United States of America

This Bramcost Publications edition is an abridged republication
of the rare original work first published in 1932.

www.BramcostPublications.com

ISBN 10: 1-934268-75-5
ISBN 13: 978-1-934268-75-9

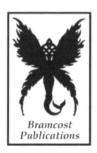

Make-up

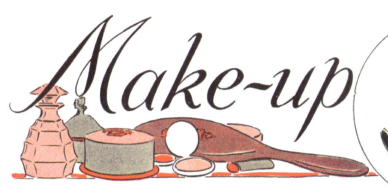

By VIRGINIA VINCENT
Author of Minute Make-ups
Illustrations by BEN ELY

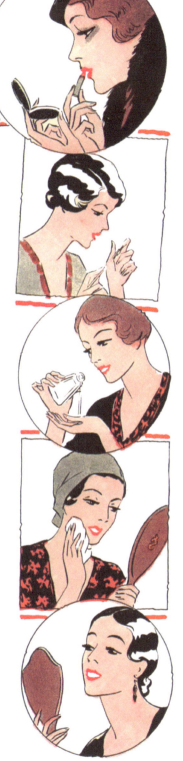

THE purpose of this book is to help you in making up your face, not according to a passing fashion but so that it expresses **you.** The following pages have been planned to help you emphasize your good features, tone down your poor ones, so that you may make your best appearance every day and enjoy the confidence which that knowledge will give you.

Begin making up your face with this book in one hand and your mirror in the other. Study your face closely observing contours and coloring. Shop earnestly for cosmetics till you have the right shades and colors. Experiment patiently in applying them. Prop this book on the dressing table and *start*— after you have followed the suggestions below.

If possible, arrange to do your make-up at a dressing table. Sitting down will relax you and takes that hurried strain from your face. Artificial lighting should come from the side of the dressing table— not from the top. The mirror should be three-sided so that you can see your own profile. There should be a magnifying mirror to use for plucking eye brows and treating black heads.

Be sure to have plenty of cotton, facial tissues and powder puffs. Stock your dressing table with small packages of cosmetics of varying shades. For your convenience, here is a list of things that you may check.

Rouge, compact, paste or cream
Powder, day and evening shades
Lipstick, day and evening shades
Cleansing cream
Astringent
   (used as directed on the label)
Pore and muscle cream or oil
Foundation cream or lotion
Hand lotion
Mascaro, liquid or cake
Eye-shadow
Eyebrow pencil
Nail bleach
Nail white
Cuticle remover
Nail polish and remover

Orange stick
Metal file
Sandpaper file
Buffer
Soap and nail brush
Pumice
Peroxide
Eyebrow brush
Eyelash curler
Shampoo
Tweezers
Waving lotion
Curlers
Perfume
Eau de Cologne

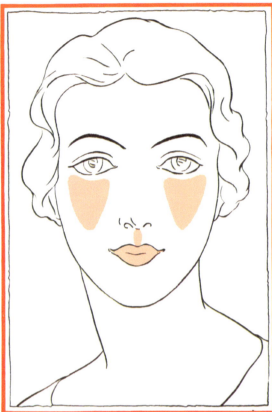

Rouge Below a Long Nose

HAVE you a long nose and a long upper lip? Your nose can be made to look shorter in a full face view by the careful application of rouge. Place a little rouge on your upper lip right under your nose. It must be a very small dab and not allowed to stray over the fluting of the lip.

Be sure to use the same color rouge that you have used for your cheeks, only do not put it on so heavily. Lipstick for your lips may be a shade brighter than your cheek rouge so that the small amount on your upper lip is hardly detectable. Paste or cream rouge will be easier to apply on the upper lip than compact or dry rouge. Do not use this make-up trick unless you are making up your entire face.

Color has much to do with changing facial contours and expressions—experiment until you get the best and most becoming colors placed to your most flattering advantage. Look at yourself critically in all lights and from all angles.

Eye-shadow on Double Chins

THIS make-up for a double chin should only be used in the evening when artificial light is particularly kind to shades and shadows. Take a little smear of eye-shadow—purplish or blue and spread it very thinly over that swell that "doubles" the chin. This won't, of course, correct the profile, but full face, it will help to diminish the appearance of the second chin.

All cosmetics should be put on over a cream foundation to look their best since much depends on their dissolving and sinking into the skin to give a natural appearance. Foundation cream or lotion should be used on the chin as well as the face before the eye-shadow is used. Powder should be used over it and great care taken that the powder matches the skin of the neck which is often a shade or two darker than the cheek powder.

In making up your chin in this way be sure to turn the artificial light on your face so that you do not make up either too lightly or too heavily. Move a lamp around in two or three positions to be sure you have achieved the effect you wished to obtain.

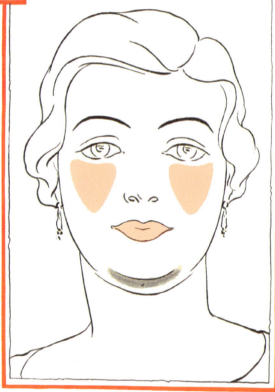

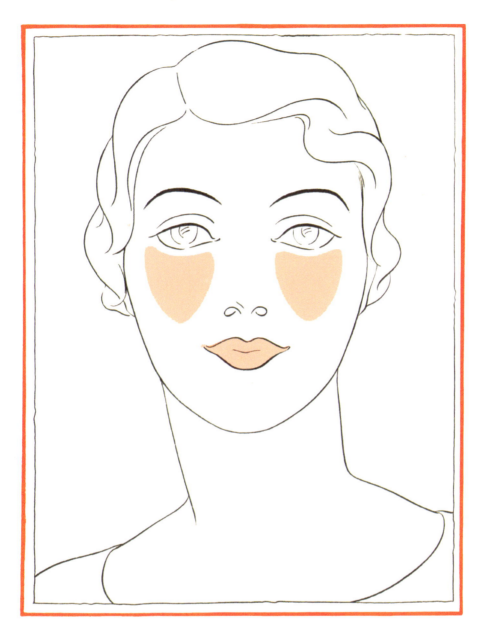

Where To Place Rouge on a Broad Face

IF YOU have a broad face be careful to place the rouge close to the nose under the eyes. It should be no wider than the width of three fingers held perpendicularly under your eye. If, by mistake, you spread rouge all over your cheeks you will find that your face will look broader than it actually is.

If you use a paste rouge, take a little on your finger and tap it lightly on the space described in the drawing above. Then blend it outward and downward, allowing the deepest color to be in the center and making it lighter at the edges. In using a dry rouge do not get too much on the rouge pad and dab it on carefully, blending it in with another piece of cotton. This will go on better if a foundation cream or lotion is used.

Remember that the rouge should be chosen with the color of your lipstick in mind so that the two blend together. The lipstick color may be brighter, but if the rouge is orange-red, the lipstick should match; if the lipstick is raspberry the rouge should match also.

Hair parted on the side rather than in the middle is more becoming to a broad face. Beware of wearing earrings that give added breadth to the jaws.

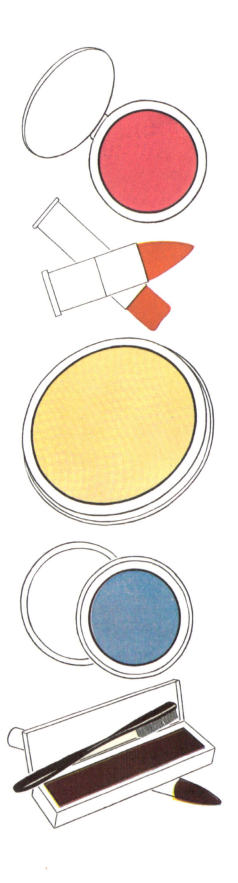

Cosmetics
For the Light Blonde

BECAUSE of the blue and white lights on platinum blonde hair, you should choose vivid cosmetics which will bring out the color of your hair, eyes and complexion.

ROUGE. You will find a bright red rouge like American Beauty will form the desired contrast with the light hair. (Rouge tints, however, for a brunette who has turned artificially blonde may have to be deeper than this particular shade.)

LIPSTICK. Lipstick must be chosen with reference to the rouge for it should vary only in intensity. The lipstick should be American Beauty, too, and used heavily. (If however, the mouth is large, beware of spreading it all over the lips.)

POWDER. You should be sure that the powder you use has enough life and color in it to contrast with your hair and give a young appearance.

EYE-SHADOW. Choose the eye-shadow that is nearest the color of your eyes. For the blue-eyed blonde blue and gray are used. For the brown-eyed light blonde, there is brown or purple eye-shadow. In the evening you may use the eye-shadow that has flecks of gold or silver through it.

MASCARO. The color of mascaro you use with this make-up depends upon the natural color of your lashes. You may wish to use a brown mascaro to match your brown eye shadow if your lashes have a brown tone. If they are black then by all means use black or blue eyebrow pencil, and black, blue or purple mascaro on your eyelashes.

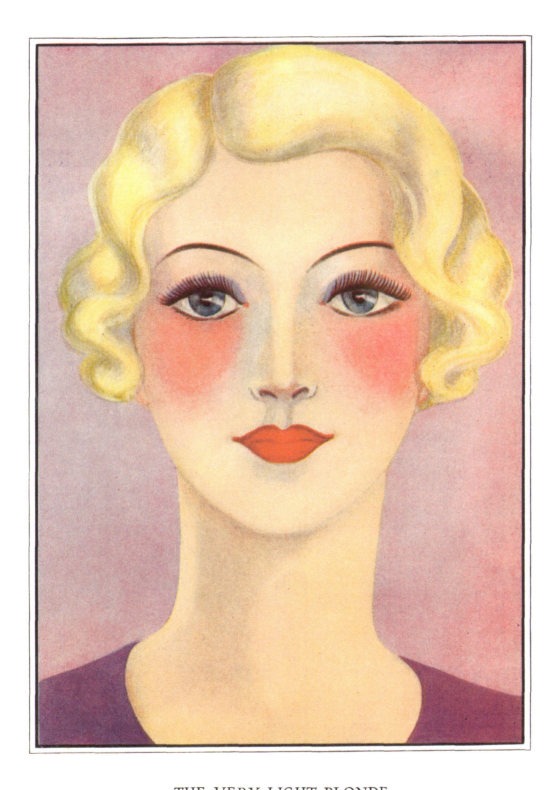

THE VERY LIGHT BLONDE

The "light blonde" is an artificial blonde. She is the delicate type and her hair, through treatment, has a bluish white color that Hollywood stars have made famous. Dark brunettes, as well as ash-blondes, have become light blondes enjoying the contrast of a dark complexion and dark eyes with the very light hair. The keynote of the light blonde make-up is contrast in powder, rouge, lipstick, mascaro and eye-shadow.

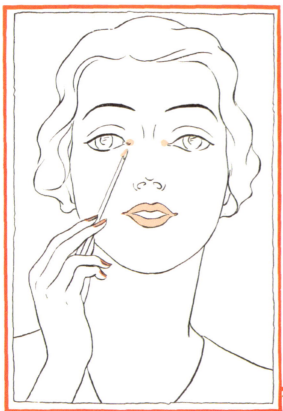

Rouge Dot at Eye Corner

IF YOUR eyes are far apart use a little round dot of rouge in each corner of the eye near the nose. The dot is almost as small as a pin head yet it lurks there in the corner of the eye to make it look bigger and more luminous.

This is how you should do it. Take a clean orange stick—one unused preferably—and dip the tip in some paste rouge of the shade that is most natural to your coloring. Twirl the orange stick in the corner till you have left nothing but a dot. If you don't hold the orange stick perpendicular it may smudge or become an oval spot rather than a little round dot. Good rouge will not hurt the eyes because the best of cosmetics are so pure that you could eat them if you liked and suffer no ill effects.

This make-up may be used for street if it is done expertly. It is best, however, under artificial light and used for evening make-up with eye shadow and mascaro. Do not use this make-up if your eyes are set very close together.

How To Groom Eyelashes

DO YOU want your eyelashes long, black, thick, curling back from the eye to make them more expressive?

They should receive as much care as you give your finger-nails. Brush them back with an eyelash brush. Smooth olive oil, castor oil or vaseline over them at night to encourage their growth. It takes 150 days to grow an eye-lash so be careful of each one and train it to grow long and curly. Constantly brushing the eyelashes away from the lid, upward, will make the lashes grow back and form a becoming fringe for the eyes to make them look larger and more expressive.

Before you acquire artificial eyelashes try to grow your own by giving them attention every night and morning just as regularly as you would brush your teeth.

To make them look darker and longer during the daytime and the evening they may be brushed with mascaro in black, brown, blue, green, purple, according to the shade that is most becoming to you.

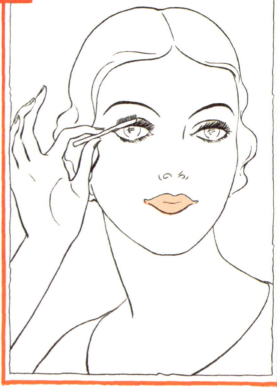

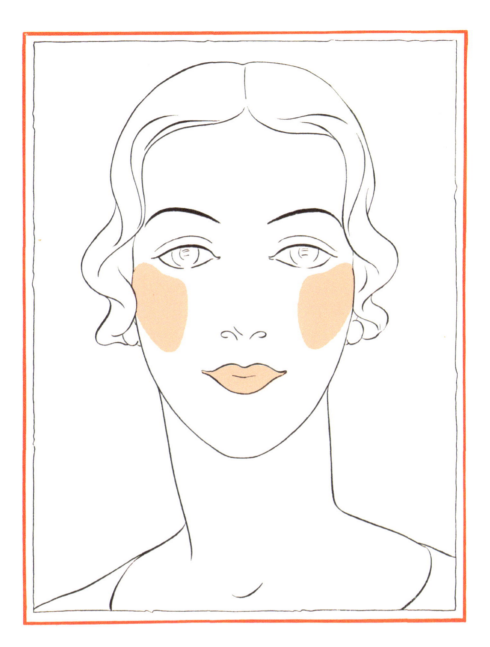

Where To Place Rouge on a Narrow Face

IF YOUR face is narrow be careful to confine your rouge to a small area around the cheek bones. Blend it out over the cheeks toward the ear to give a broadening effect to the face. Do not let it spread toward the nose as that has a tendency to make the face look long. Rouge kept well out on the cheeks will also make a sharp or oval chin less pointed.

You must take care that you get the rouge on evenly or the effect will be lost. Rub the rouge pad, if you are using compact rouge, in a circle at the edge of the cheek, then carefully spread it up and down. If you are using the paste or cream rouge, pat a little on the cheek bones and coax it in a circle so that the color fades out toward the edges just as natural color would do.

Be sure not to use a white powder on your nose because it is apt to make it appear prominent and therefore lengthen the line between your forehead and your chin. Use a powder that will blend with the rouge and your natural complexion and which is not noticeable in the brightest daylight or under artificial light.

Parting your hair in the middle will also do much to give a broader effect to your face.

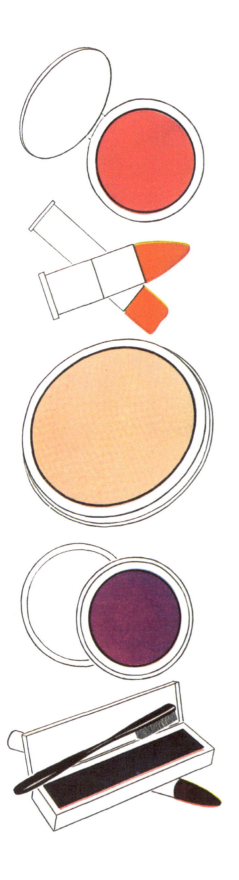

Cosmetics
For the Golden Blonde

THE most striking thing about the golden blonde is her hair. It should have frequent shampoos to keep its color, becomingly arranged to show its sheen, and have dress colors chosen to reflect its glory.

ROUGE. If your skin has the natural creamy quality, a rose-colored rouge or a geranium both having yellow in them, will blend very naturally with it. If your skin is more white than cream you may need to select a rouge with more orange in it.

LIPSTICK. This should be a different color than the rouge—much more than one or two shades brighter. A cherry color you will find the best and most becoming shade.

POWDER. You may want to use rachel or an ecru powder, but this will be more becoming if it is a rose-rachel to carry out the pinky tints that are the charm of most blonde complexions.

EYE-SHADOW. Because golden blondes vary so greatly in the color of eyes, you will find that the most becoming eye-shadow is probably a mixture of two colors—one put on over the other. Try blue and gray with the blue predominating. Or peacock green and blue with the blue the strongest color.

MASCARO. The eyelashes may be quite interesting if blue mascaro is used to make the eye-shadow more pronounced. The eyebrows ought to be darkened with brown eyebrow pencil if they are too light.

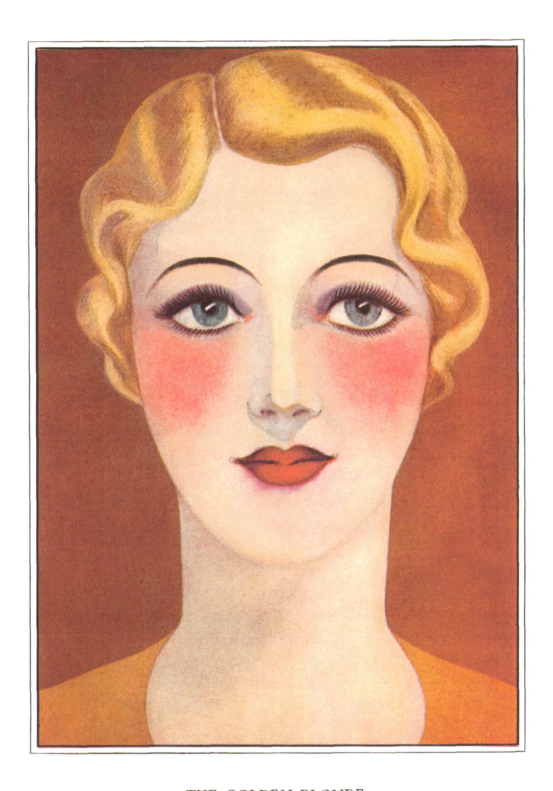

THE GOLDEN BLONDE

Has your hair golden blonde colors in it? Have you blue, violet, hazel or gray eyes? Have you a fair complexion? Then you are a blonde. Blonde colorings will never be monotonous if the right cosmetics are used to deepen the natural colorings and to accentuate the creamy fairness.

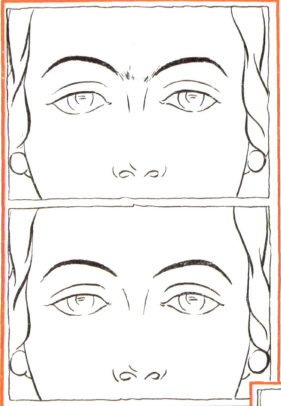

Allow One Inch Between Eyebrows

OBSERVE your eyebrows in a magnifying mirror. Are there any little hairs that bridge the space over your nose and make the eyebrow a continuous line? Sometimes this gives the effect of frowning when otherwise the face as well as disposition is serene.

There may be a few stray eyebrows or the eyebrows may grow too near together. Take a pair of tweezers and sit down before your magnifying mirror and go to work to jerk them out one by one. Pluck out all these misplaced hairs that make a continuous eyebrow line and see how your expression changes. There should be between three-quarters of an inch and an inch space between the eyebrows.

Take a tape measure and measure before you pluck them. Notice when you are finished how much more delicate the bridge of your nose appears. See the beauty it gives to your brow. If you keep these hairs plucked they will grow in slower and slower and, in time hardly at all, so that you will have less and less work to do in plucking them.

The pictures at the left show the eyebrow before and after it has been plucked over the bridge of the nose.

Tidy Up Your Eyebrows

HAVE you fuzzy or shaggy eyebrows? Eyebrows should not grow down to on the concave side of the eye socket. Nor should eyebrows grow in peaks and points toward the forehead.

Take your magnifying mirror and your tweezers and decide what line and width you desire to have them. (Don't **ever** use a razor to shave them nor scissors to cut them off in a hurry. Clipped eyebrows are decidedly ugly looking.)

With your tweezers pluck out the hair that straggles up on the forehead or low toward the eyelid. If in plucking the skin becomes sensitive take a little witch hazel and dab the eyebrows with it before proceeding. Have patience and take only one hair at a time and be sure not to pinch the skin else you will have a tiny swollen pore the next day.

Take great care not to pluck too many so that you have an artificial look. If you have naturally heavy eyebrows allow them to be heavy and keep them in line through plucking the straggling ones on each side.

This picture at the right shows eyebrows before and after they have been trained by plucking and brushing.

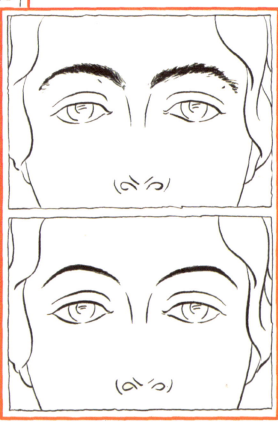

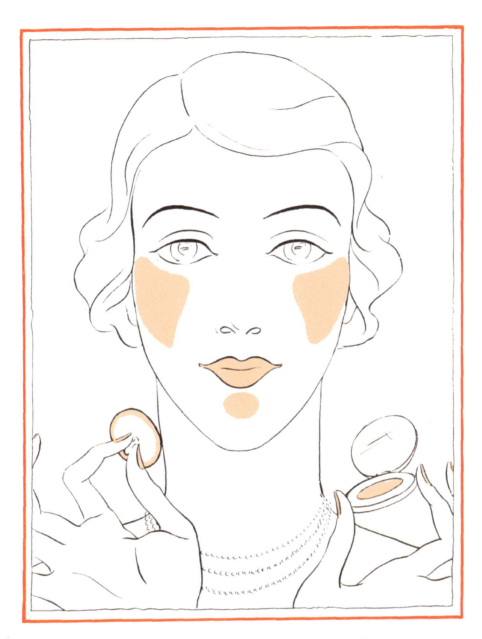

How To Place Rouge on a Long, Oval Face

HAS your face long lines? Is it oval rather than round? Is the chin pointed instead of square? Then, when you make up, follow these suggestions in placing rouge on your face. Put your rouge far out on your cheek bones blending it outward toward the ears and keeping it well away from the nose. Be sure the heaviest color is under the eyes and far out on the cheek.

Put a small dab of rouge on your chin—do not apply it nearly as heavily as you did on your cheeks. The rouge on your chin will give your face a much shorter appearance and the rouge far out on the cheeks will make it appear wider. Rouge coming directly under the eyes makes them look larger and more luminous. If you have hollows in your cheeks be sure not to allow the rouge to go over them in such a heavy manner that it accents them. Keep it high on the cheek bone and use a powder that will blend with the cheek rouge so that the transition from no rouge to the part of the cheek that is rouged will not be so sudden as to be noticeable.

As in all other make-up, if you prepare your face by using a cleansing cream and astringent you will find that the rouge will give bloom to your complexion instead of a "painted" look.

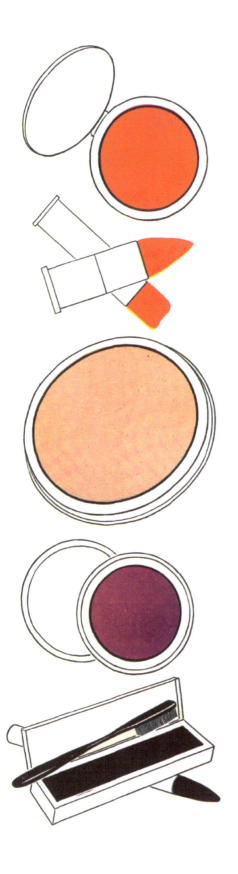

Cosmetics
For the Chestnut Brunette

YOU may not resemble exactly the chestnut brunette in coloring of eyes and hair, but in using cosmetics you can follow the general shades of rouge, lipstick, powder, mascaro and eye shadow illustrated on this page.

ROUGE. This shade of rouge has a slight bluish or purplish cast. The exact shade whether it should be deeper or lighter will be determined by the dark tone of your complexion. Only by experimenting with rouges of this shade can you find out which is best for you.

LIPSTICK. The lipstick is deeper than the rouge for the cheeks and should be definitely a deep Cherry color.

POWDER. Most brunette complexions look best with a blend of rose and rachel powder. Try matching the powder to the skin in the hollow of your shoulder which is said by beauty experts to give you the key color to your complexion.

EYE-SHADOW The eye-shadow may be purple or green according to the color of the eye. Try them both and see which is most becoming. If you have brown eyes the purple shadow proves the most becoming.

MASCARO. The eyelashes for the brunette are most striking when brushed with a black mascaro. For an alternative use a deep purple like the eye-shadow. The eyebrows may be touched up with brown or black eyebrow pencil.

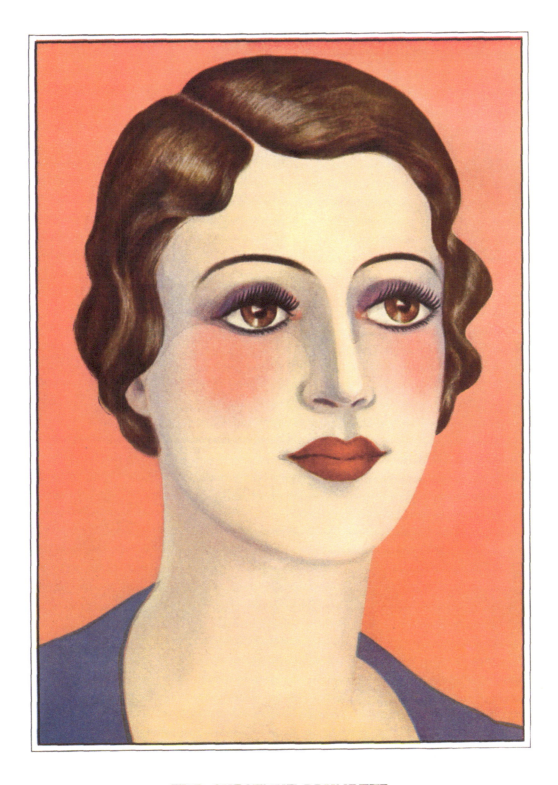

THE CHESTNUT BRUNETTE

If you have dark eyes, you are a brunette. The chestnut haired brunette with dark eyes may have a fair skin but the cosmetic colors should be chosen for her brunette coloring. She may use hardier colors in cosmetics than the blondes just as she effects the sharper greens, reds and purples in her costumes.

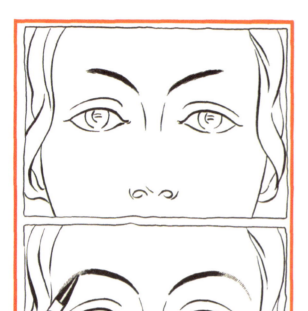

Pencil Out the Eyebrow Line

HAVE you the too delicate type of eyebrow that does not curve completely to the corner of the eye?

This kind of an eyebrow does not bring out the contour of the brow or make the eyes as effective as they should be.

If you cannot grow more eyebrows by using vaseline and oil applications take an eyebrow pencil that matches your eyebrows in color and extend the line of the brow where it would naturally grow. Carry out the arch of the brow carefully, keeping the line as thick as your natural eyebrows and making the line light enough so that it is hardly detectable even in your own mirror.

Notice how your expression changes and your face gains in width. Eyebrows are very important because they govern the expression of your eyes.

How To Train Eyebrows

IF YOUR eyebrows are unruly and apt to get out of alignment, train them to stay in place and grow together by brushing each eyebrow with an eyebrow brush.

Wiry, bristly eyebrows may be softened by using soap on the eyebrow brush or by smoothing them with vaseline. You must use your eyebrow brush carefully, first brushing them down from the top toward the eyelid. Then brush them out toward the temples so that each lash is in alignment.

Those who use mascaro on their eyebrows should be sure to remove it at night—softening them with cream or ointment because mascaro has a tendency to dry the skin. Eyebrow pencil is best to use to darken the eyebrows and should be in dark brown or dark blue according to the tone of the eyebrow. Blondes usually use the brown, brunettes the blue.

Be sure to brush the powder out of your eyebrows after powdering even if you are not using any make-up on your brows.

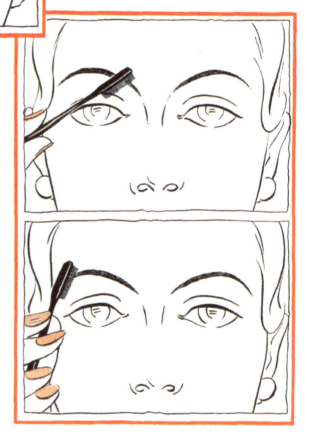

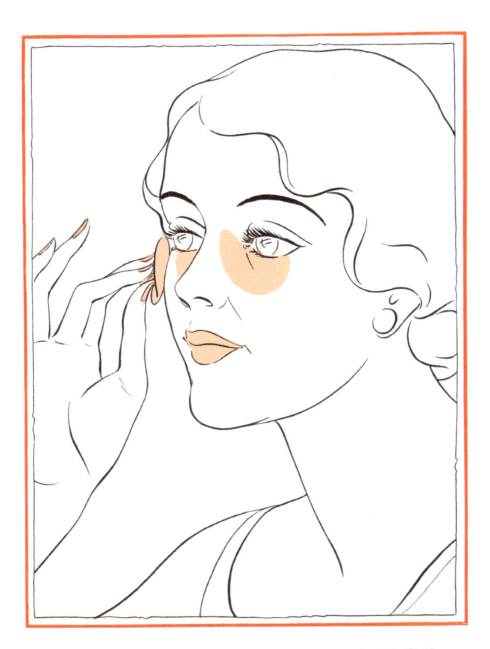

How Rouge Is Applied for a Youthful Effect

THE placing of rouge as illustrated above is the trick of a famous French make-up artist. For those who are over thirty years old it works wonders in erasing the marks of time. To get the best results forget about the regular rules of rouging.

First prepare your face with a foundation cream or lotion. Then take the right color rouge according to your natural coloring and place the rouge directly under your eyes and up, well up the side of your nose. Then extend it under the eye to the extent of about two fingers placed parallel to your nose. The rouge so close to your eyes makes them sparkle and deepens the color.

The powdering is important with this make-up. You need two shades. One quite pinkish and deeper in color than your usual powder for the cheeks, the other fainter in color for the chin and neck. The powder with the pinkish or rose tone gives the cheeks a delicate coloring and should cover the rouge that is placed on the side of the nose and under the eyes. Eyeshadow and mascaro should be used effectively with this make-up.

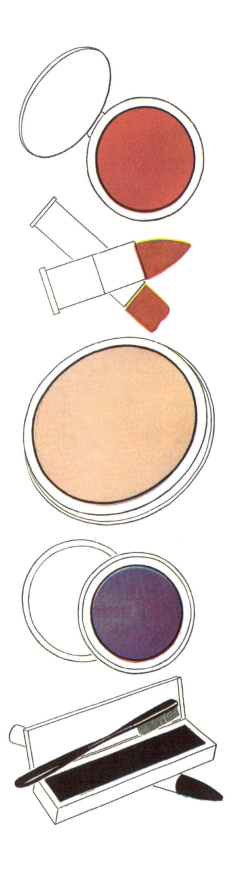

Cosmetics
For the Spanish Brunette

THE very dark brunette may be daring in her make up, especially if her eyes and hair are inky black. If your skin has the lovely olive texture you may omit the rouge on your cheeks and simply make up eyes and lips.

ROUGE. If the skin has a dusky shade, a raspberry rouge may be used. Shade it carefully and lightly into the skin as if you were an artist painting a water color.

LIPSTICK. The lipstick is brighter than the rouge but with the same bluish-red cast.

POWDER. If your complexion has a deep dusky cast, use a powder that will blend with it. It may be necessary to use two shades of powder—one heavier on the cheeks, another creamier for the neck.

EYE-SHADOW. If you have black eyes or very deep brown ones, purple eye-shadow will prove most effective.

MASCARO. You should use black mascaro for the eyelashes, brushing both the lashes to the under eyelid as well as the lashes to the upper eyelid.

EYEBROW PENCIL. If the eyebrows need widening or lengthening use a black eyebrow pencil. Do not apply it too heavily. You may need to use it to extend the line of the upper eyelid at the corner to make the eye look bigger.

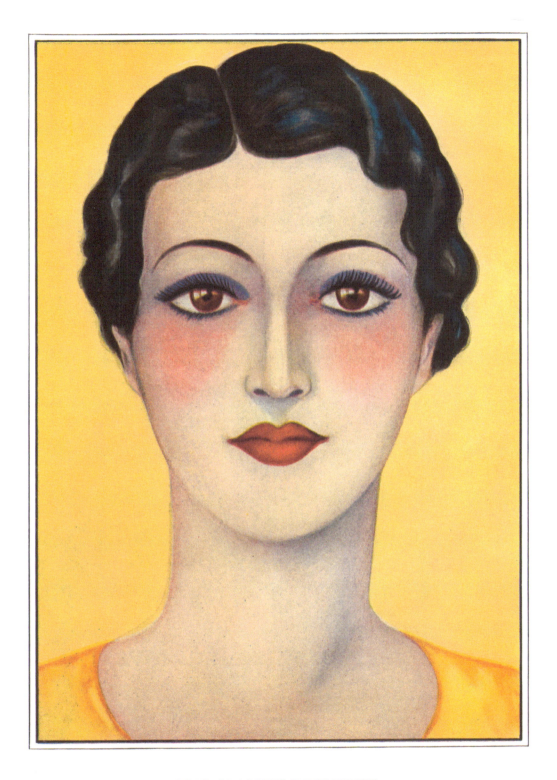

THE SPANISH BRUNETTE

This black haired, dark eyed type of brunette has either a deep rich swarthy complexion to be made up as described on the opposite page or a magnolia skin which is most striking if only the lips and eyes are made up. If you have this coloring, choose the raspberry reds in rouge, the deep ruby colored lipstick colors which are considered "old" for any other type of beauty.

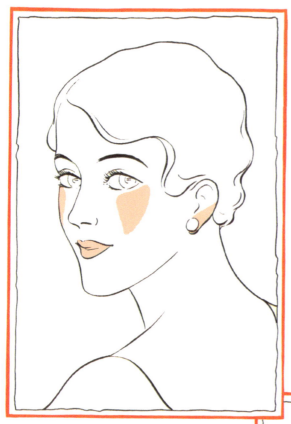

Rouge the Ear to Give Width to the Face

DOES your face have better proportions when you add width to it? If the jaw line is oval and the nose long, arrange your hair to show your ear and rouge the lobe of it.

Use the same rouge you are using for your cheeks only apply it more lightly so that your ear takes on a shell pink tone. (If you make it too red it will look frost-bitten.) Paste or cream rouge will be easiest to use on your ear.

Be sure if you wear ear rings to wear the button style rather than the long drop fashion. Button ear rings will make your face look wider instead of longer. The arrangement of your hair near the cheek bones will also give a broader effect than if you drew it down over your ear.

Don't Accentuate the Jaw Line

ARE you sure that you rouge properly? Do you confine the rouge area to the upper part of your face indicated by the dotted line in the picture at the right?

Often rouge seems to slide down lower on the face accenting the jaw line and making it look heavier than it is. Rouge placed low in the cheeks also makes you look older because it gives a drawn expression to the face.

Those who have prominent jaws should avoid using heavy lipstick or rouge. The best effect is often gained by using two kinds of powder, one for cheek and one for chin so that the cheeks and the cheek lines are emphasized rather than the lower lines of the face.

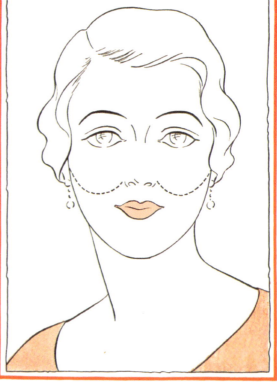

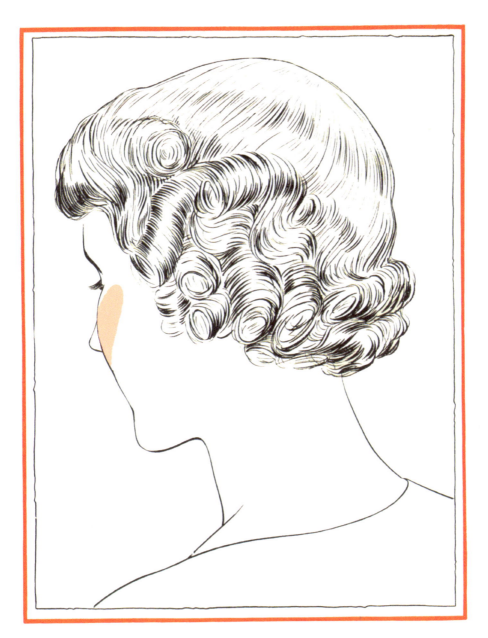

How To Wear the Curly, Longer Bob

THE curly long bob is being used by those in their teens and twenties and those who wish they were still at that age. It is especially attractive with the small hats or sport bandeaux.

To accomplish this effect you should have your hair very simply waved about the face and the longer hair waved in spiral curls. Be sure that it is long enough because the curls will shorten it considerably.

Notice that the curls are spiral or round curls, quite different from the usual marcel wave. You can get this effect by winding the hair on kid curlers or using a curling iron.

If you want the curl to stay in the hair, use a little brilliantine on your brush before you start curling. Tying your curls carefully in place under a hair net at night will help them set and make them last longer than they otherwise would.

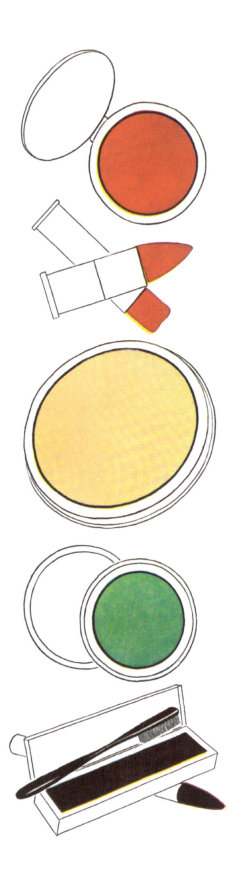

Cosmetics
For the Light Red-Haired Type

THE new colorful cosmetics have made make-up far more effective for you who have auburn hair. There are at least 15 shades of rouge, one of which is particularly suited to you.

ROUGE. Be sure your rouge is geranium and that it is on a definite orange-red tone. Do not apply it heavily because it will look artificial over the white skin, often freckled because it is so sensitive.

LIPSTICK. You should match your lipstick to the rouge but, of course, it will be brighter as you will use it more heavily. Do not be afraid of a contrast with your hair because a lipstick of this color should simply harmonize the color of your lips to your hair.

POWDER. The powder should have a yellow cast—not at all like the powder used by the light blonde. It should be ochre with a tint that is known as nude.

EYE-SHADOW. Use green eye-shadow by all means. It is flattering to hazel eyes, brown eyes, or green eyes.

MASCARO. The eyelashes should be deepened by a brown mascaro and the eyebrows by a brown eyebrow pencil.

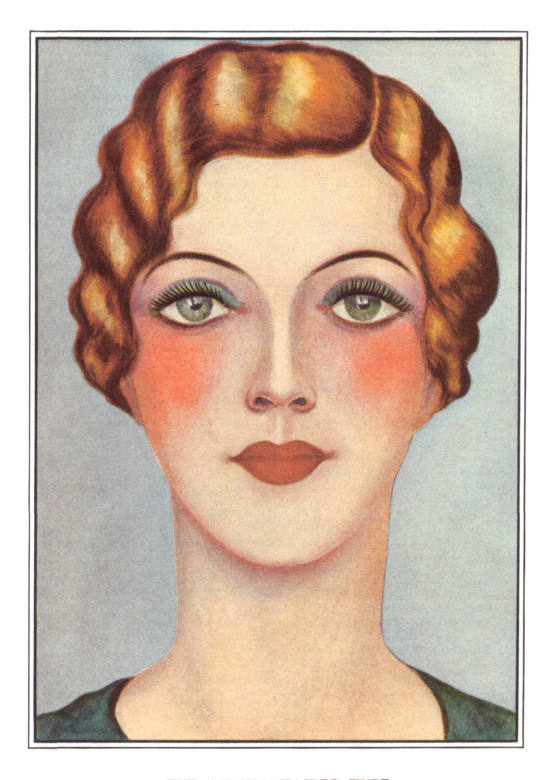

THE AUBURN-HAIRED TYPE

You who have light red hair will find make-up a necessity, because your hair is so colorful that it over shadows the natural coloring of face and eyes. Because of the brightness of your hair, the cosmetics used will also be more vivid. The white sensitive skin so usual with red haired people needs particular attention in the matching of powders both as to color and texture.

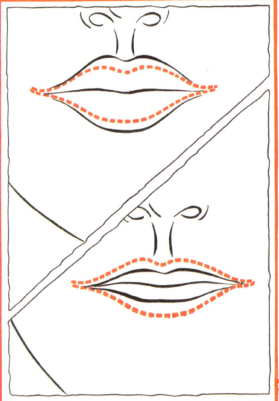

Less Lipstick for Full Lips

IF YOUR lips are wide or full do not spread lipstick to the outside edges. Curve the lipstick below the lip-line and notice how much smaller and thinner the lips appear. To reduce the size of the lips use two color lipsticks. The heavier color on the upper lip and the lighter color on the lower lip. Full lips should never have too much lipstick on them. Close your lips over a piece of facial tissue and allow it to absorb the excess amount if you wish to give them a thin covering of lipstick.

More Lipstick for Thin Lips

If your lips are thin and show only a narrow line of red, you should use more lipstick spreading it slightly over the outer lip-line. Be sure to match your cheek rouge with your lipstick. Take the natural color of your lips as a guide for selecting the color you should use. Allow lipstick to dry on your lips thoroughly and it will last longer.

Extend the Eyelid Line

A LONG eyelid line will add greatly to the expressiveness of your eyes. Extend this line by using an eyebrow pencil at the outside corner of your eye. The pencil should be used lightly and then blotted with your finger tip so that the line lingers vaguely under the powder. This makes your eyes look larger.

Eye-shadow for Emphasis

Eye-shadow is used on the upper eyelid to give it contour and to bring out the color of the eye. Eye-shadow—and it comes in all colors—should be put on with the tip of the finger along the lower part of the eyelid so that there is contrast between the lid and the skin under the eyebrow. Sometimes a slight touch of vaseline instead of eye-shadow may be used on the eyelid to give a "moist" appearance and accentuate the curve of the lid.

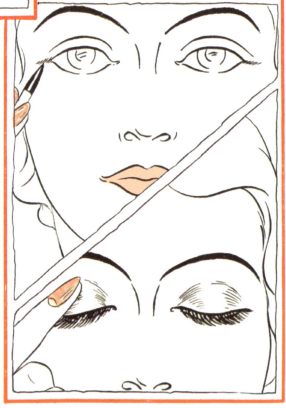

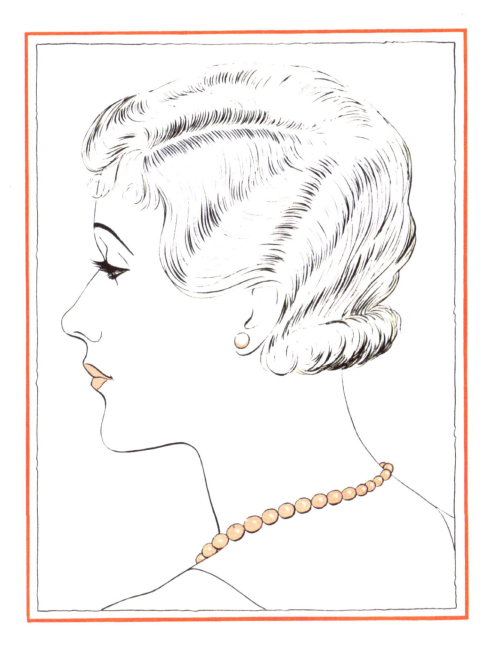

Suit Your Coiffure to Your Profile

BEFORE you decide on your hair arrangement sit before a three sided mirror and scrutinize the shape of your head, the profile of your nose, the height of your forehead, the outline of your ear.

If you have a well shaped head the coiffure above may suit you. The roll at the nape of the neck is made of the growing bob or a similar arrangement may be effected by pinning a transformation from ear to ear. The flat effect and the ears showing is becoming to many broad faced or full faced people. The curls on the forehead are easily made by using a waving lotion and pinning the hair in curls with invisible hairpins.

This is the natural coiffure to use when your hair gets longer than a short bob and shorter than long hair. It may be kept in place by a barrette and invisible hairpins. This is a simple coiffure for those with natural curly hair.

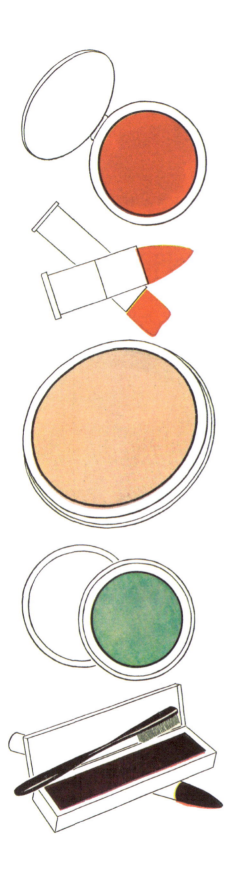

Cosmetics
For the Titian-Haired Type

CHOOSING cosmetics to go with red hair has always been considered a problem since it meant the blending of the reds of rouges and lipsticks with natural red hair.

ROUGE. You will find a carmine rouge which, in the hand, may look entirely too red but the minute it is applied, the color blends in with the skin and gives a natural coloring that contrasts with the color of the hair to make it still more beautiful.

LIPSTICK. Don't be afraid of a scarlet lipstick. This lipstick should be carmine and applied not so heavily that it looks artificial, but so skillfully and thoroughly as to make the lips quite red and tempting.

POWDER. Don't shun pink powder either. This powder should be more nude in tone than pink but it should have the skin tone so that the face when well powdered takes on a healthy glow. You may have to mix the powder yourself, blending two kinds of powder, one with pink and one with yellow in it.

EYE-SHADOW. Green eye-shadow looks best with the particular color of eyes that go with red hair. For evening you may want to use the green or purple eye-shadow with the glints of gold in it.

MASCARO. Eyelashes look best with brown mascaro brushed on them—never bead them with mascaro but brush them the length of the lashes. You may brush the eyebrows with the brown mascaro or use a brown eyebrow pencil to make them darker.

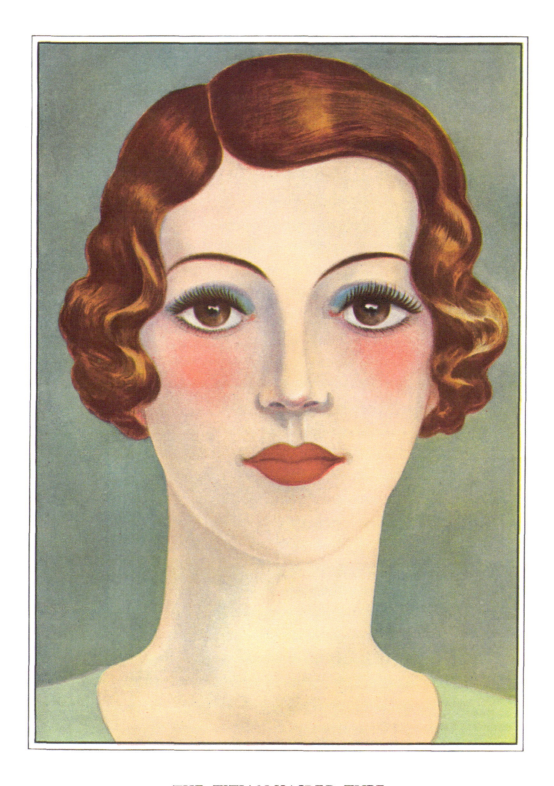

THE TITIAN-HAIRED TYPE

You may call the color of your hair Titian, or henna or plain dark red—any of these shades denotes a particular type of beauty that is most difficult to make-up. Eyes with this color hair are often brown, golden brown, hazel, gray-green—so that a blend of two colored eye shadows are better than one. The color of rouge and lipstick varies with the color of hair so that infinite care should be taken in order to get the right tone.

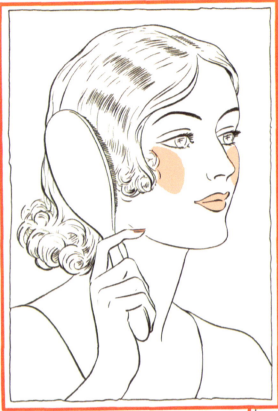

How To Use Brilliantine

BRILLIANTINE is used to make the hair more manageable after a shampoo and also to give it added sheen and a pleasant fragrance. It is excellent for making fine hair look well groomed and for controlling stubborn, fuzzy ends. Put a drop of liquid brilliantine or rub a little salve brilliantine on the palm of your hand. Then rub your hair brush over it. Be careful not to get too much brilliantine for then it makes the hair look oily. Brilliantine acts best on dry hair.

Even though brilliantine helps to set a wave on newly marcelled hair do not neglect to brush your hair thoroughly night and morning. Brush vigorously up and down, toward your face and away from it because that is the best way to stir circulation and keep your hair so healthy that it is naturally glossy and colorful.

Can you pinch your scalp between your thumb and index finger? If not, massage it with your finger tips so that it becomes flexible and you will see an improvement in the color texture and handling of your hair.

Rouge for Elbows and Hands

ARE your elbows white or darkish in color? First rub a little vanishing cream around your elbow bone till the skin is soft and smooth. Then take rouge, either paste, compact or cream, and apply it lightly on each side of the elbow bone.

This will give the dimpled effect that is youthful and very charming. While this is not strictly make-up for the evening it is most effective when a decollete gown is worn.

If the palms of your hands are colorless, use rouge on the inside finger tips and the thumb and on the little mounds below each finger across the palm. If the rouge does not blend into a "pink," use a slight application of liquid powder. Hands should look as young and delicate inside as they do outside. This is a theatrical trick used under the bright lights of the stage and must be done very subtly if your hands are to be seen under the light of a bridge lamp dealing cards.

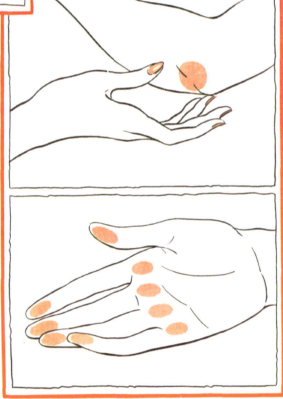

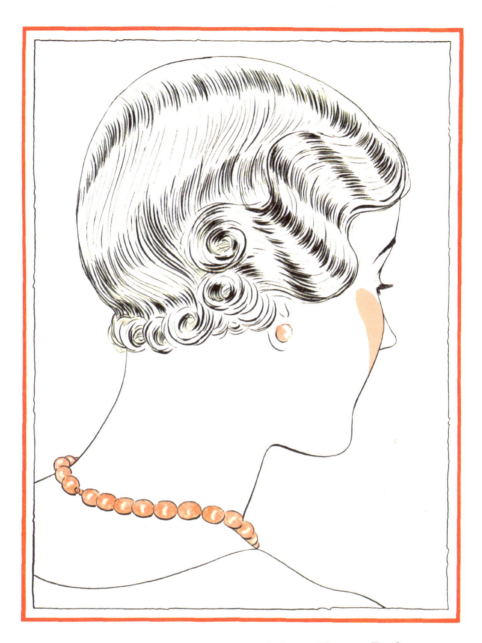

Another Variation of the Short Bob

IF YOU are tired of short hair, change your bob! Look at the hairline in the back of your neck and decide if you would like the effect of long hair along the back of the neck given by these short curls.

You must have at least two inches of hair at the back of your neck with which to make the curls. This hair should be permanently waved if you wish it to stay in place neatly. Invisible hair pins will do much to keep the curls in shape after a shampoo especially if a waving lotion is used.

The sides of your hair should be long enough —you may have to have it thinned—to be pinned back over the ears. If the hair is thick it will flop toward your face and spoil the close smooth effect which makes a short haired bob look like long hair. The back of the head is kept straight—unwaved and unswirled—with the hair combed down from the top of the neck to the neckline where the little round curls are arranged.

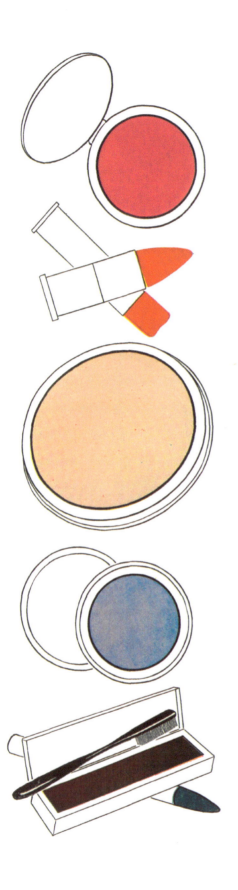

Cosmetics
For the White-Haired Type

THE colors you select for costumes is no clue to the colors you select in cosmetics if you have gray or white hair. You should strive for contrast with your hair by selecting bright, young colors in cosmetics.

ROUGE. The rouge may verge on the raspberry shade having a slight old rose tinge. It should be put on very skillfully so that it blooms on the cheek instead of "spotting" it. It may often be brought high on the cheek bone and near the hair line at the temple.

LIPSTICK. You will want a brighter lipstick with less of the bluish color that is associated with the sample of the rouge above. Lipstick will be carmine and not applied too heavily.

POWDER. Since blondes and brunettes both have white hair, you must choose the color powder to match your skin color. Be sure, however, that it has enough of the dark pinkish tone in it. The blonde-gray types will find this powder very youthful in effect.

EYE-SHADOW. The color of the eye-shadow should be blue or purple for the gray-blonde (see illustration) and for the gray-brunette, brown or dark green may be used.

MASCARO. Eyebrows and eyelashes are very important as they should be directly in contrast with the hair. The eyebrows may be darkened with black eyebrow pencil. The eyelashes may take their tone from the eye shadow used. To have blue mascaro on the eye lashes to match the blue eye-shadow adds greatly to the effectiveness of the eyes.

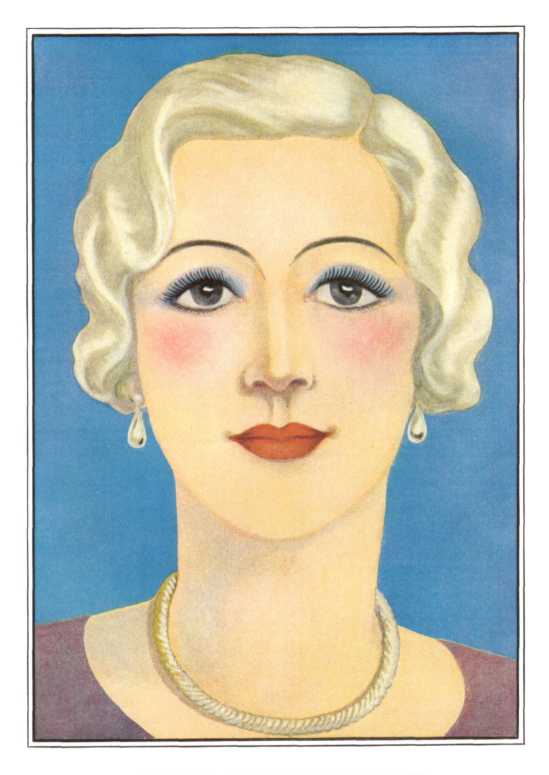

THE GRAY- OR WHITE-HAIRED TYPE

There are two types of women with gray hair. Those who have young faces and gray hair and those who have older faces and gray or white hair. The make-up for both is nearly the same except that those who have won their gray hair through added years should use cosmetics less generously than those who have a more youthful complexion. Like the light blonde, the white or gray haired woman should choose her cosmetics for the effect of contrast.

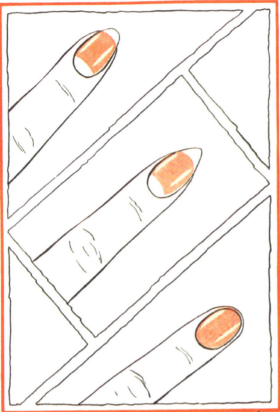

File Your Nails According to Your Finger Profile

BEFORE manicuring your nails determine which one of the three following types of finger nails will make your hands look most attractive.

If you have a medium length finger, shape your nails in the almond shape allowing a small amount of the white of the nail to show. Almond shaped nails are considered the most ideal type. If your fingers are short you may like to use the very pointed nail to make them look longer. To have the nail extend a half inch or longer from the finger tip is the popular talon fashion.

If your fingers are very long and also if the nails are brittle use the short round nail that barely comes over the finger tip. This is particularly practical for office and home workers who have trouble with broken nails. Brittle nails should be nourished with applications of olive oil or castor oil.

The most beautiful well groomed hands should show nails with a half-moon at the base. This can be developed by carefully and constantly pushing the cuticle down with an orange stick. This should be done gently otherwise the nail will be bruised and will be marred as it grows with white spots.

To Keep Nails Looking Clean

IF YOUR nails get stained or have a tendency to look dingy despite frequent cleaning, you should use a nail bleach.

One of the easiest ways to bleach your nail "whites" is to use a white manicure pencil with a point that may be run under the edge of the nail. The point of the pencil should never be so sharp or run so deep that it hurts the cuticle. Another way to bleach your nails is to run a bleaching manicure cord under the edge of the nail. Do this before you use an orange stick to clean your nails. The cord must be wet so that the bleaching powder sticks to the under side of the nail.

Bleaching should be done after the nails are filed with a steel file. A sandpaper file may be used afterwards to smooth the edges if necessary. If bleaching dries the cuticle, go around the nail with an orange stick wrapped in cotton which has been dipped in olive oil. Cuticle removers may be used for a nail bleach effectively if the nail is not stained badly.

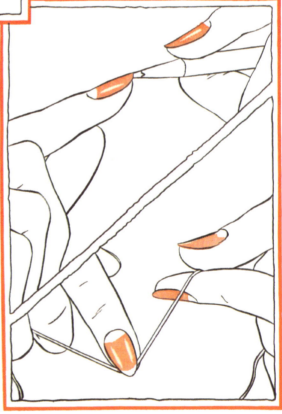

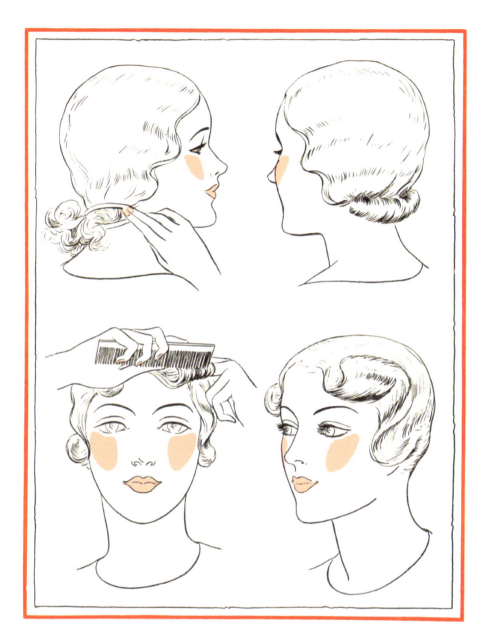

How To Arrange Hair of Awkward Length

DO YOU wonder how to keep hair of awkward length so that it is tidy and has that well groomed look? If you have hair that is at the "in-the-neck" length use a curved barrette at the nape of the neck to hold all the short hairs firmly in place. See head, left top. The hair is brought over and rolled, pinned firmly in place with hair pins until it looks as smooth and neat as the head at the right.

Have you short hair on your temples that flops over when you bend and which disarranges your long hair? Perhaps you should have it thinned, and cut so that it can be trained to swirl back to meet your long hair.

Try to do this training yourself by placing your index finger on your hair close to the head and comb your hair over it as pictured. This will allow the ends to curl back to the rest of the hair as in the next head. This is much used by those who effect the more severe type of coiffure. Invisible hair pins will help greatly in training your curly locks to stay in place.

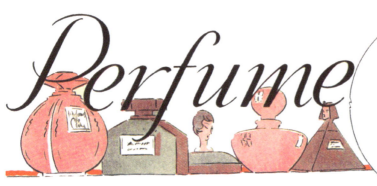

Perfume

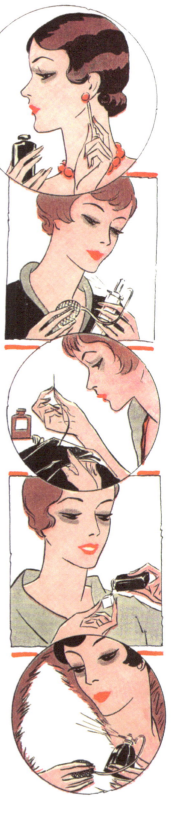

NO ONE should purchase a perfume because it is fashionable or because she admires it on some one else. The perfume that suits a blonde will not suit a brunette nor a scent that is meant for a vivacious outdoorsy type of person will not be becoming to a studious, languid individual.

The selection of perfume is almost entirely intuitional and must be chosen because you "feel" it is right and not for any other reason. Price does not enter into consideration for an inexpensive perfume may suit you far better than an expensive one. The best way to make your decision is to get a small bottle of a scent that you think you are going to like and carry it around with you. Does it fit in with your moods? What is the reaction of other people to it? Does it belong to you?

For day time wear, consider the single flower scents. The rose, lily of the valley, violet, gardenia, sweet pea, verbena, lilac, heliotrope, mimosa, and lavender. For evening wear, you may think of the Oriental scents, musk, chypre, special bouquets and mysterious and fascinating mixtures defying recognition.

If your perfume bottle has a glass stick in the stopper, touch the ear lobe with it. At the same time you can rub this stopper around the hair line at the back of the head. This gives the hair a fragrance.

Use an atomizer to spray your neck and shoulders with perfume. This is the most economical way to use perfume as it is distributed evenly and lightly over a greater area. (It also, if used on a dress, prevents it from making stains or spots.)

If you wish your clothes to have a faint scent, put a drop of perfume on an old kid glove (the kidskin will retain the scent) and sew it into the hem or the seam of your dress. Do you want a sweet breath? Saturate a lump of sugar and eat it before you go out to an evening party.

Your furs should have a delicate fragrance. Spray them with perfume an hour or two before you go out so that the perfume evaporates and the fragrance clings to them.

Perfume lingers longest if applied directly on the skin. For some reason it also adheres to woolens whereas it vanishes quickly on silk and cotton. Remember this when you use your atomizer.

Printed in the USA
CPSIA information can be obtained
at www.ICGtesting.com
JSHW040922250824
68635JS00002B/8